Save the Girls
Cancer Became a Victim of My Praise

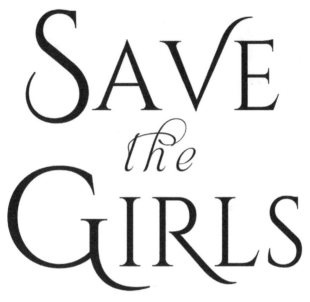

SAVE *the* GIRLS

Cancer Became a Victim of My Praise

YOLANDA PERRY

XULON PRESS

Xulon Press
2301 Lucien Way #415
Maitland, FL 32751
407.339.4217
www.xulonpress.com

Unless otherwise indicated, Scripture quotations taken from the King James Version (KJV) – *public domain.*

Printed in the United States of America.

ISBN-13: 978-1-54565-397-5

DEDICATION

Dedicated To Dr. Wanda Hatter-Stewart, my beloved physician who worked at Family Christian Health, Harvey IL. She believed and prayed with me that God would bring me through my breast cancer journey.

TABLE OF CONTENTS

FOREWORD

Yolanda has documented her personal healing journey
with breast cancer using her own unique perspective
and narrative, and in doing so, shares how faith and
spirituality are so integral to the experience of a cancer
diagnosis and treatment. By sharing her emotions and
vulnerabilities, and surrendering them to a higher power,
she is a role model of what human strength and resiliency
can be like.

Eugene Ahn MD

Consistency.
I admire consistency.
Yolanda Perry is consistent.
She is one of the most consistent people I know.
She is consistent in her love for her family and friends.
She is known to be remarkably consistent in her walk
with our Lord.

This book details her journey from a dark and forbid-
ding place to a season of light and great possibility. In this
book, you will read of her seasons of heartache and tears.
Yet, you will also have a chance to see into the great heart
of a woman of remarkable faith.

This may seem to be an unusual observation, but I believe Yolanda displayed remarkable patience while working her way through this process. The Word "patience" is actually a shortened version of "patient endurance."

I believe my translation of Luke 21:19 describes this victorious season of Yolanda's life. "It is through your patient endurance that you save your own life." She patiently endured, held onto the promises of God and came out the other side of this thing better than when she went in.

Read this book.
Highlight this book.
Make this your warfare manual.
Make it more than reading material.
Use it as a weapon against ill health.
Above all, use it as a resource to build your faith.
Yolanda's journey proves we are never really alone.
If you're suffering, in the Name of Jesus, I call you whole.
"Faith is the victory that overcomes the world," (1 John 5:4).
Your faith is working for you, and you will have your desired result.

Most Sincerely Yours,
Malcolm Burton, Th.D.
Madison County, Texas.

INTRODUCTION

Approximately five years ago, I supported a young lady who had been diagnosed with cancer. I ventured to her home and prayed with her and her family, visited her in the hospital, and showered her with encouragement. At the time, I never thought I would be the one diagnosed with breast cancer. Thanks be to God, I was surrounded by a gracious and loving family and supportive friends who showered me with their encouragement, time, and prayers.

My journey with breast cancer began when I received two annual mammogram-reminder cards mailed to me in June and July of 2016. Given that my annual checkup was already pre-scheduled for August, I pondered on whether or not to go in for an earlier annual mammogram. During this time of contemplation, I was encouraged by a nurse to schedule an early annual mammogram.

After my initial mammogram appointment, I received a call from my doctor's office to come in for a second mammogram screening. I informed my pastor, his wife, and my mother of the possibility that I might have breast cancer. I'll never forget the love and support I received from each of them. My mother called every day of the week to check in on how I was handling the process. And my pastor's wife attended my first biopsy appointment with me. As I recall, she arrived at the doctor's office well before I did, and sat there with her Bible on her lap, praying and waiting. As I've already mentioned, I never thought I would be the one diagnosed with cancer.

In August of 2016, my family gathered to celebrate the seventy-eighth birthday of my grandmother, Mary Patterson. After the event, I decided to share my diagnosis with my family. As the family convened around the dining room table, I informed everyone that I had been diagnosed with breast cancer. Tears streamed down my face as I explained the intricate details of my diagnosis. My family was indubitably supportive. Two of my cousins Tremayne and Taiwan, stood by my side, one with his arm on my shoulder and the other gently caressing my hand. Their support gave me strength and hope that I could only garner from a loving family. I will never forget that night. As a family, we cried and prayed together. Afterward, the family agreed that for every radiation visit a loved one would attend with me. I was truly blessed to have nineteen loved ones attend every radiation appointment with me. The prayers and support of family and friends far and near contributed to my victory over breast cancer.

As you read about my victorious quest over breast cancer, I pray you will be inspired, transformed, and healed. My prayer is that you are blessed by my journey to victory over breast cancer. My girls were saved, and breast cancer became a victim of my praise.

LIFE WITHOUT CANCER

Tuesday, July 12, 2016: The Call to Prayer

My periscope notification for Pastor Hannah woke me up for his 4 a.m. prayer call. That morning Pastor Hannah challenged everyone to pray for the next fifty days at 4 a.m. I accepted the challenge, and I asked my mother to be my prayer partner.

At the time, we had no idea that those fifty days of prayer were preparation for what was to come next. Almost immediately following the completion of the fifty days of prayer, I was diagnosed with Ductal Carcinoma in Situ (DCIS). DCIS is a non-invasive cancer where abnormal cells reside in the lining of the breast's milk duct.

Wednesday, July 13, 2016: Recognizing the Miracles of God

First Miracle - I attended my annual mammogram before my pre-scheduled date.

Second Miracle - I received a fee waiver for a new mammogram test called Tomosynthesis - 3D.

When I checked in for my annual mammogram appointment, the receptionist explained the difference between an annual mammogram and a 3D-Tomosynthesis mammogram. The receptionist gave examples of the differences between a traditional mammogram and "Tomosynthesis- 3D Mammogram."

A traditional mammogram depicts images of the first layer of breast tissue. It's similar to looking at the first slice of a loaf bread. A Tomosynthesis 3-D mammogram encapsulates images of several layers of the breast tissue. This is similar to looking at a loaf of bread from the side to review each slice of bread.

The Tomosynthesis 3-D mammogram was not covered by any insurance in Illinois, therefore, there was a fifty dollar fee. This fee was waived by the mammogram office. To God be the glory!

When the technician called me in for the Tomosynthesis 3-D mammogram, I noticed that there were more images taken of my breast than usual. Although I was not nervous, I was curious about why this was so. Despite the unusual amount of images taken of my breast, I had peace and was not worried about the test results.

Friday, July 15, 2016: Patience is a Virtue

When I called my doctor's office to receive my results, she had not completed the reviewable process.

In the meantime, I received a call from the mammogram office on July fifteenth stating that I needed additional testing, and that my doctor's office would be giving me a call with my Tomosynthesis 3-D mammogram result.

After receiving the news from the mammogram office, I immediately called my doctor to inquire information on my test results. I was informed that the review process had not yet been completed. On one hand, I had no idea of the outcome from my Tomosynthesis 3-D exam. And on the other hand, the mammogram office informed me that I needed to come in for additional testing.

I called my mother and informed her that I needed additional testing and requested that she attend my next appointment. We agreed not tell anyone what was going on. Maybe it was because I chose to believe I did not have cancer until I was told differently. Maybe it was because I was expecting God to change the situation. Maybe I was just scared.

Sunday, July 17, 2016: Love and Compassion

During praise and worship service, my pastor's wife laid hands on my right breast and prayed for me. Then she spoke words of encouragement.

Monday, July 18, 2016: The Report

Finally, I spoke with my doctor, and she informed me that calcification was found in my right breast and fibroids in my left breast. Breast calcifications are small calcium deposits that develop in a woman's breast tissue. They are very common and are usually benign (non-cancerous). Even after receiving the news, I continued to believe God that all was well. I allowed the peace of God to rule in my heart, and I refused to worry about anything. During this time, my mother faithfully called me on a daily basis to uplift my spirit.

Thursday, July 21, 2016: Second Mammogram

I received my second mammogram and ultrasound of my left breast. During this round of testing, I had peace. The care and service from the staff was exceptional; they even permitted my mother to witness the ultrasound procedure.

Sunday, July 24, 2016: Praising God

In spite of the process, I continued to praise. I was determined to give God all the praise and honor despite what the doctors said, the images showed, and what the test reported. My praise was a powerful weapon, even during the waiting process.

Tuesday, July 26, 2016: Biopsy

My pastor's wife joined me for my biopsy appointment. She arrived early once again and was ready to intercede on my behalf. She spoke gracious words of encouragement and prayed for my well-being.

Fortunately she works in mammography, so I received the best quality of care. I was allowed to see the breast tissue that was removed. The tissue looked like the fat you remove when cleaning a chicken. The dye that was placed on the sample turned the calcified tissue blue.

I continued to believe in God for a miracle and that all would be well despite the results. The staff kept me informed every step of the way.

This was a mentally heavy day, but I chose to trust God and continued to believe all was well.

Wednesday, July 27, 2016: Quality

I received a call from the biopsy doctor, she inquired about how I was doing. She made me feel important and shared with me that she had not yet received my test results. She informed me that immediately upon receiving the pathology report, someone would call me with the results.

I was yet praising God in spite of the wait. I refused to worry about my results and believed God that all was well.

Thursday, July 28, 2016: Commitment & Miracles

During the two weeks described above, I was preparing a Prayer Focus for Dr. Cassandra Scott Ministries (CSM). I was scheduled to submit the focus by Wednesday, July 27, 2016.

However, I did not submit the Prayer Focus until Thursday, July 28, 2016, for the Monday, August 1, 2016 to Friday, August 3, 2016 presentation.

During my personal prayer time, I meditated on Ephesians 3:20. While reading the book of Ephesians, this verse had pricked my heart and spoken loudly to my spirit. Later that morning, my mother prayed Ephesians 3:20. I praised God for Ephesians 3:20 and decided this was the focus scripture.

I proceeded with the Focus preparations. The Focus was "Created to Produce Supernatural Results." The prayer focus scripture was Ephesians 3:20, "Now unto Him, that is able to do exceeding abundantly above all that we ask or think, according to the power that worketh in us..."

The daily topics were:
Monday - Power of God
Tuesday - Faith
Wednesday - Preparation
Thursday - Suffering
Friday - Results "Signs and Wonders" and "Spiritual Humility"

I chose to speak on Wednesday, August 3, 2016, but had no idea that I was also scheduled to meet with the general surgeon to discuss preparations for cancer removal on that same day.

After presenting the prayer focus, I began to concentrate on my health. Eventually I was not active in CSM; I was no longer a leader of a prayer team, and I became an inactive administrator.

On my way home from work, I received a phone call at approximately 5:30 p.m. from my primary care physician. This was startling because she never called me after 5 p.m. Following a cordial greeting, she asked me if I was sitting down. I informed her that I was driving. My doctor stated she had my test results, and I needed to schedule an appointment to see her.

Third Miracle
I informed my primary care physician that I had an appointment with the obstetrician/gynecologist (OB/GYN) doctor on Friday, July 29.

Fourth Miracle
The doctor scheduled me as her first patient for that day.

After, speaking with my doctor, I immediately called my mother and told her I believed that the doctor was going to give me some bad news. She encouraged me stating, "No news does not mean it is bad news."

Refusing to worry about what news I would receive, I called and texted my pastor and his wife to let them know about my appointment. I continued to believe God that all was well.

DIAGNOSIS

Friday, July 29, 2016: Good & Bad News

Second Appointment Cancelled
First Appointment Cancelled

I arrived at the OB Doctor's office and my appointment was canceled because the doctor was out of the office. While waiting for my primary doctor, I listened to CSM Prayer Line on my cell phone speaker. When I registered for my appointment the doctor's staff stated, "We heard your prayer call. Please keep us in your prayers," and I agreed.

Friday, July 29, 2016, Continues

I mentioned that we could say a prayer after my doctor's appointment with the doctor's approval.

Second Appointment

My doctor entered the room. She explained that she had good and bad news. The good news was if there was a form of cancer to select from this would be the best one to choose.

It was Ductal Carcinoma In Situ (DCIS). Now the bad news was that I had cancer. My response was, "There's an anointing that will be released upon my life from God." I had a positive attitude, and I wanted God to get the glory from my testimony.

I remembered to call my mother so that the doctor could share the news. After she told my mother, I praised God as I remembered He is able to do exceeding abundantly above all we can ask or think according to the power that works in us, (Ephesians 3:20).

I was ready to be used by God in prayer. I requested to pray for my doctor and the staff. The doctor's staff entered the room with us. We all held hands before I led the prayer. I praised God for the opportunity to pray, and I claimed all their souls for the Kingdom of God.

<u>On my way to work: Mentally Processing the News</u>
I began to contemplate if I wanted to tell anyone that I had cancer. While pondering on this decision, my mother called and asked me to tell my brothers. She could not carry this any longer without letting anyone know. I agreed to tell them on Saturday, July 30.

Then I stopped at Wendy's order a Combo one with a single cheeseburger, fries and frosty for emotional eating and as comfort food. I called my friend and shared with her that I have been diagnosed with cancer. I truly wanted to believe God for a miracle and to not have to receive any form of treatment. I once again was thinking about what the family wanted and not want I truly wanted. My friend and I talked about natural remedies, wellness centers, and various books about alternative medicine. I had not made a decision and limited my conversation about my discernment for no medical treatment (radiation/chemotherapy).

Friday, July 29, 2016 Continues:

Work/Weekly Prayer and Meeting
I led the weekly prayer at work. I prayed that God's will be done in our lives. No one knew that I had been diagnosed with Breast Cancer. I continued to allow God to use me and prayed for others. By the choice of my will, I prayed and praised God in spite of the diagnosis.

Then I met with my supervisor and shared the news with her. We discussed my leave of absence, vacation, and sick time. It was amazing as I was thinking about whether or not to share the news with my children, my boss advocated for them. Therefore, I decided to tell them after I picked up my son from school on that upcoming Wednesday, August 3.

On my lunch break, I attempted to contact my roommate, my pastor, and his wife. I left them all messages notifying them that I had been diagnosed with cancer. I texted my roommate, and she called me. We briefly talked and arranged to speak to a cancer survivor that afternoon.

After Work: Mental Processing Continues
While driving to get my oil changed, I heard the scripture John 11:4 in my spirit: "...not all sickness is unto death." Awaiting the completion of my oil change, I had a three-way call with my roommate and a breast cancer survivor. She suggested I focus on my healing and to be in tune with the leading of the

Holy Spirit. She also suggested that I be in prayer regarding who to share my diagnosis with. During this time, we prayed and praised God, and I was strengthened.

Saturday, July 30, 2016: Brotherly Love

My sons and I ventured to Southern Illinois University to pick up my daughter from college for summer break. After arriving home, I met with my brothers to announce the breast cancer diagnosis.

As I explained the information to them, I began to cry. This was the first time I had cried since my doctor told me I had cancer. After telling my brothers, the eldest brother stated, "I knew it."

The middle brother shared a scripture God have given him, John 11:4,

"When Jesus heard that, He said, this sickness is not unto death, but for the glory of God, that the Son of God might be glorified thereby."

God is amazing. That was the exact scripture God had given me on Friday. When my brother shared the verse, I considered that to be a confirmation from God that all was well. This confirmation from God provided me with the strength to continue to have faith in the word of God and to trust Him through this journey.

Love of My Children: Sharing with my Youngest Children

On Wednesday, I was scheduled to have a meeting with my three children. However, there was a conflict with my daughter's work schedule, so my mother and I met with my two youngest children to share the news with them. My youngest son reacted with anger and a willingness to fight if anyone spoke ill of me. Then he encouraged himself by stating "My mom is not going anywhere." When my daughter left for work, she called her best friend and cried, and they comforted her.

Sunday, July 31, 2016, Morning

Love of My Children: Sharing with my Oldest

My eldest son and his family come over to my Mother's place. I informed my eldest son and his wife of my diagnosis. They both reacted to the news by crying. My mother and I comforted them letting them know we are trusting God to bring us through. Informing my eldest son was a very emotional and sensitive moment. My son and his wife had previously supported my daughter-in-law's mother who is also a breast cancer survivor. I could not even imagine how they felt. Before my diagnosis, they were both enrolled in college but decided to postpone their education to attend my doctor appointments with me. Words cannot express how blessed I was to have their support.

Sunday, July 31, 2016, Evening

<u>Family Gathering - Sharing with Extended Family</u>
My family celebrated my grandmother's eighty-seventh birthday. As I was contemplating on whether or not to inform the family of my diagnosis, my mom asked me, "Are you going to tell the family?" I decided to inform the family after the celebration had ended and after my grandma had left.

I was glad my grandma decided to leave the party early as I did not want to ruin her celebration. When I shared the news with my family that night, all my cousins were present with the exception of four.

As I was sharing, I began to cry for the second time. My two male cousins came and stood by me, one on each side. I told them that it was worth having cancer if this caused all of us to draw closer to God.

This was a wakeup call for our family. I expressed to them that I was standing for our family in prayer. My prayer was for each of us was to continue to develop a personal relationship with God and for their marriages to prosper. I decreed and declared that every marriage connected to our family tree would prosper and that my marriage would be the last divorce in the family.

After I spoke with everyone, I had the opportunity to elaborate on their feelings. That night each family received prayer and a word of encouragement. It was truly a blessed night.

Monday, August 1, 2016: Not in Denial

I sat up in my bed and said to myself, "I am not in denial; I know I have cancer, but yet I believe God for His will to be done." I began to praise God for who He is. I decided that God's goodness was not predicated upon the outcome of this situation, that God was good in spite of my diagnosis.

The question of the hour was, "Are you moving home with your mother?" Yes, I moved back home with Mom on August twelfth, so she could further support me as my caregiver.

Wednesday, August 3, 2016: Preparation

<u>CSM Prayer Focus</u>
This day started with presenting the focus for CSM's prayer call. The topic was "Preparation." I felt as if this was such a divine timing for the topic to be preparation. I was the speaker for the CSM call, and I spoke about preparation for the supernatural experience of God. And I was attending my pre-op and general surgeon doctor's appointment in preparation for surgery to remove the calcification tissue from my breast. The topic was preparation, and I attended my preparation doctor appointment.

Pre-op Appointment

I attended my prep-op doctor's appointment. The staff thanked me for praying for them on July twenty-ninth. My doctor encouraged me and said she expected me to do well through the process. Then we prayed before I left the doctor's office.

General Surgeon Appointment

I asked if my support team (two sons, my mother, and room-mate) could come with me into the exam room. The nurse put us in the largest room. The doctor pulled the curtain shut and conducted the breast exam. He explained the surgery process and answered my questions. I asked the doctor if He believed in God. He replied, "Yes." I shared with the doctor that I was believing God for a miracle, and that yes, I hoped for the miracle that no cancer would be found.

He stated, "Let me share with you what I define as a miracle:
1) You're a good patient that got your annual breast exam.
2) The cancer was detected early.
3) The procedure will be a success.
4) You will complete your treatment and be healed."

I replied, "You are not in agreement with me?" My roommate intervened by stating, "You both believe in miracles."

I leapt off the table and stated, "Let us pray!" I grabbed my doctor's hand and began to pray. He appreciated the prayer I prayed. I believe in the Word of God. The Scriptures state if two touch and agree in my name it shall be done (Matthew 18:19). I prayed for a successful surgery, the surgery team, and my miracle.

Love of My Children - Sharing with My Son

My mother and I went to pick up my son from college. My brother and my sons met us at my mother's place. I shared the news with my son. He was very emotional. He thought I was going to die.

I informed him that I was not dying and it brought him comfort to know. He stayed with me twelve of the fourteen days he was home from school.

Thursday, August 4, 2016: Testimony & Words of Encouragement

I had spent the week facilitating the CSM Morning Prayer Call. That day's topic was suffering and my mom was the speaker. It was an honor that she agreed to speak. The call was powerful, and I shared my story. I encouraged all callers to attend or schedule their annual mammogram because they save lives. I even shared with them that on Wednesday, the topic was Preparation and I attended my Preparation appointment to have the cancer remove.

I continued to stand in faith, believe in God, and give Him the praise in the midst of this situation.

Friday, August 5, 2016: Oncology Appointment I met with the oncology doctor. He informed me that DCIS cancer is not life-threatening. If it spreads, it still would not be life-threatening.

After the removal of the cancer, the following will be my treatment options:

1) No further actions to be taken.
2) Take a pill for five years to suppress the estrogen in my body.
3) Radiation if the cancer spreads.

The doctor informed me that my tissue would be tested by the hospital and forwarded to a lab in California to determine how my body will respond to radiation and chemotherapy. The lab tests would be used in determining how much radiation or chemotherapy would be needed to administer in the event such was necessary.

I was in good spirits and still believing in God for a miracle. The doctor answered all questions, and I yet believed God.

Monday, August 8, 2016 - Sunday, August 14, 2016: Leading up to Surgery

This the first time my roommate and my children were at home at the same time. This was the week I had to deal with reality. I had unresolved feelings about my children. I was preparing to move home with my mother. I was mentally preparing for the surgery on Friday, August 12.

Work/Perseverance

This week, I only worked Monday and Tuesday. It was difficult to focus on paperwork and filing documents into clients' folders. I did my best to concentrate. I informed my boss on the status of my files. I was able to have everything in sequential order. The doulas would be able to service clients after reviewing my documentation if needed. I informed my boss that I had a client due any day. I prayed that she would not have her baby until I returned to work on August 22, 2016.

Work-Family Sharing with Staff

I was very hesitant about sharing with management and colleagues. I wanted to share with them when I was ready. I also wanted them to hear the news from me and no one else. At those earlier times, I was not ready.

After, discussing my decision with my supervisor, I informed my doula colleagues that I would be taking some time off work and may need coverage for a birth.

They were concerned, and I assured them everything was ok. Due to me taking days off for appointments; my colleagues had joked about I will be at work on Monday, Tuesday, and Wednesday and then off on Thursday, Friday, and Monday.

We would laugh and joke about when I would and would not be at work.

Family Time - My Children

I enjoyed spending time with my children. I was disappointed because we planned a family outing to Great America, and I was not able to attend the family outing because I was recovering from surgery.

Therefore, I encouraged my children to attend the family outing without me. They made plans for their outing. I became overwhelmed with all my children and my godson being at the apartment Wednesday night and Thursday morning. I realized Thursday morning that I was still serving my children, preparing breakfast, cleaning, and fussing. They even attempted to put me out of the kitchen as they prepared breakfast but I refused.

Suddenly, I realized that I did not like being rejected. Consequently, I lived to please my children. I failed to correct and discipline them when I should have. My lack of discipline caused problems in their lives. Their teachers complained about their lack of respect. Moving forward, I realized that I could not fear rejection. I must now be their mother and sister in Christ. I must demand respect as I endured this season of my life.

Wednesday, August 10, 2016: Starting Preparing for Surgery

I was very emotional, stressed, and needed a clean bedroom as I cleared my mind. My children organized their belongings before leaving the house. I was able to rest. While I was resting, I remember sitting up in the bed saying, "I am not in denial." I was present to the fact I was diagnosed with cancer.

Honestly, I desired to be alone for the next two days but that did not happen. I took this opportunity to examine my emotions. Then I examined and processed my emotions with my roommate.

Then I wrote a list of everything I regretted about my life. During this moment, I cried until I stopped and went to sleep. My roommate heard me crying and eventually checked to make sure I was ok. Before I realized it, the day was gone and only one of my children returned.

Thursday, August 11, 2016

Everyone agreed that it was best for me to live with my mother during my cancer treatment. All day I packed my belongings in preparation to move to my mother's place that evening. I prepared dinner: macaroni and cheese, fried chicken, cornbread, and cabbage. This was a very special dinner for me because this was our family time before my next day's surgery.

Afterward, we walked to the lakefront and released pink and blue balloons in memory of a family member. I was very emotional as we released the balloons, prepared for surgery, and left my roommate. We had become as close as sisters.

I knew it was time to depart. I had a brief conversation with my roommate. Then we transported my belongings into the car. As we traveled to my mother's place, I became overwhelmed. I began to cry. I did not allow my children to see me crying. I cried silently as the tears rolled down my face and met underneath my chin. I thought, "Tomorrow my body will never be the same again." God blessed me to acknowledge my feelings and yet believe in Him through the process.

THE PROCESS

Friday, August 12, 2016

This was the day of my surgery. I am so grateful to have a supportive community (family, church family, and friends). As we walked through the same day surgery unit, the staff stopped their work and looked at us. One staff member stated, "She has a lot of support." My four children, daughter-in-law, and mother were with me.

Everyone entered the room until they had to leave for my preparation. Once the nurses prepared me for surgery, everyone returned to the room, including my pastor. Everyone was laughing and talking as we waited for me to be transported to surgery. Then the nurse entered the room. She explained to my family that they have to wait in the family waiting room until I returned.

Surgery

Step 1:
I was transported to the MRI department for testing. DCIS is not visible to the natural eye therefore, an MRI test was conducted on my right breast.

Step 2:
I was transferred to the radiologist's room. The radiologist conducted a procedure called wire-localization. I was not numb

during this procedure. This was a painful procedure. I was instructed to squeeze the nurse's hand. I was disappointed no one had mentally prepared me for this procedure administered with no pain medicine while a wire was being inserted into my breast.

The radiologist used the breast MRI as a guide and inserted a very thin wire into the breast. Then blue dye was injected into the areola area for the lymph nodes procedures. Then I was transferred to the surgery waiting room. While I was waiting to be transferred to the operating room, my mother and my dear friend were permitted to visit me.

Fifth Miracle
While they were with me, the surgeon informed me that I was next for surgery. He also said, "This is the first time in my career that I've been ahead of schedule." I was informed later that my friend prayed with the surgeon before she returned to the waiting area.

Step 3:
The surgeon then used the inserted wire as a guide to find and remove the DCIS. About 7.5 centimeters (equivalent to the size of a baseball) of my tissue was removed from the breast area. Three lymph nodes in the underarm area (axillary nodes) were removed to check for cancer cells. After the surgery, I was transported to the Same Day Unit.

I requested to be admitted overnight and the nurse refused. My dear friend of twenty years was the only person who was able to wake me up to go home. I was on bedrest from Friday, August 12, 2016, until Friday, August 19, 2016.

Tuesday, August 23, 2016: Report

I attended the follow-up appointment with the surgeon. He informed me the DCIS had spread beyond the milk duct. The treatment he recommended was definitely radiation but said the oncologist may recommend chemotherapy. I was disappointed, I wanted the report to be no cancer found. Yet I trusted God to carry me through the process. I continued to thank God in spite of the report.

Thursday, August 25, 2016: Options

I met with the oncologist to discuss my plan of treatment. The oncologist ordered an Oncotype test to determine treatment. He explained two plans of treatment.

The first would be radiation and hormone therapy for five years.

The second plan of treatment would be chemotherapy once every three weeks for six treatments, Herceptin one year, radiation five weeks, and hormone pill for five years. My heart would be monitored every three months. The oncologist and I discussed me receiving a second opinion on Thursday, August

31, 2016. We agreed to further discuss my plan of treatment when I returned on September 8, 2016.

Thursday, September 8, 2016: Final Decision

The oncologist recommended a year plan with Chemotherapy, Radiation, Hormone Therapy, and Herceptin medication. I told the oncologist that the second doctor had recommended the same treatment plan. Then I revealed to the oncologist that I was going to Cancer Treatment Center of America for my treatment.

REFLECTION - LOOKING BACK

Events

I took the time to process my emotions. I only talked to my children, brothers, and spiritual leaders.

I was disappointed because I did not have the testimony that I desired. I wanted the testimony that the doctor removed the breast tissue and no cancer was found. I appreciated the fact that the cancer was detected early. I reflected on the process:

1) June 29, 2016: I was diagnosed with DCIS.
2) August 3, 2016: I went to doctor appointments:
   a. Primary doctor pre-operation appointment for surgery clearance
   b. General Surgeon doctor appointment
      i. We were not in total agreement. I was believing God for a supernatural miracle (that no cancer be found).
      ii. The doctor stated the miracle was already present. The cancer was detected early.
      iii. We agreed that we both believed in miracles.
      iv. I prayed with the surgeon and my family before leaving his office.
   c. Surgery was scheduled for August 12, 2016
3) Successful removal of DCIS on August 12, 2016
4) August 23, 2016: I was informed I needed further treatment.
5) August 25, 2016: Additional tests ordered to determine treatment plan.

I wanted a second opinion before the surgery on August 12, 2016. I thought my family would be angry with me if I delayed the surgery. Therefore, I did not reschedule the surgery. Instead, I scheduled an appointment for a second opinion. The first available appointment that was August 30, 2016.

During this time, I appreciated the women of God who were in my life. I shared with a dear sister in Christ the care I was currently receiving. I was receiving weekly chiropractic adjustments. In addition, I went to a Naturopath for cholesterol screening with oil supplements.

I also met with a nutritionist to review my diet. Honestly, I was overwhelmed by trying to keep so many doctors informed.

My dear sister encouraged me to contact Cancer Treatment Centers of America (CTCA). She recommended CTCA because of their reputation for developing individual treatment plans for their patients. The CTCA treatment plan would include all of my services delivered under one roof, instead of several.

Spiritual

On July 12, 2016, my mother and I began to pray at 4 a.m. At the time, we did not know I would be diagnosed with DCIS. We continued to pray and thank God for the journey and made preparation. I chose to believe in God for a miracle. I realized that God was able to perform miracles. God could miraculously heal me. I continued to praise and worship God. I knew that I was in a win-win situation.

To be out of the body is to be present with God. God assured me that I was not dying from cancer. He confirmed it with the Word of God. "All sickness is not unto death," John 11:4.

I began to reflect on my life and realized that I had unforgiveness in my heart. The process of forgiving began as God revealed to me whom to forgive.

No man knows the heart but God. I realized that my testimony will give other men and women hope. "We overcome by the blood of the lamb and the word of our testimony," (Rev. 12:11).

My testimony will make a difference in people's lives. In order to be healed, I had to forgive others. By the choice of my will, I chosen to forgive people for hurting and disappointing me.

SECOND AND THIRD OPINION PROCESS

Wednesday, August 31, 2016

Second Opinion
I attended the appointment for my second opinion. The mammogram tech conducted a mammogram screening. She reviewed my medical records (mammograms, biopsy, and surgical reports) from my primary care doctor.

The first and second doctors recommended the same two treatment plans. The second doctor's final recommendation would be given after the pathologist reviewed my twenty tissue slides. They also wanted to conduct the BRCA1 and BRCA2 gene test. The BRCA1 and BRCA2 gene test is a blood test that can tell you if you have a higher risk of getting cancer. The name BRCA comes from the first two letters of breast cancer. I did not schedule the BRCA1 and BRCA2 gene test.

There was a battle in my mind. Positive and negative thoughts continue to come. Meditating on the Word of God was my strength. Remembering John 11:14 comforted me.

Later, the second hospital staff member called me with good news. The pathologist reviewed the slides and recommended radiation only.

The feeling of relief overtook me. Praising God was mandatory. On this day, I was approved to schedule my third opinion at Cancer Treatment Center.

Tuesday, September 13, 2016 - Thursday, September 15, 2016

Third Opinion
An early morning appointment was the beginning of my day at CTCA. I was overwhelmed by attending various doctor appointments. It took three days of testing to develop a unique, individualized care plan. I met with nurses, genetic consultants,

three different oncologists (medical, radiation and gynecological), naturopathic medicine, nutrition consultant, chaplain, and survivorship.

The oncologist ordered a MammaPrint test to determine a treatment plan.

The radiologist stated I should only need radiation therapy. The oncology gynecologist evaluated the fibrous tumors in my uterus. The purpose of the evaluation was to rule out uterine cancer and to determine if I needed a hysterectomy.

Once my evaluation was complete, chiropractic services and massage therapy were added to my care plan. It was a blessing to be offered a care plan with all services (body, mind, and spirit) at one location.

Finally, my decision was made to continue my journey at CTCA. Words cannot express the feeling of alleviation.

Counseling

The literature from the hospital recommended that I attend a counseling and breast cancer support group. On Thursday, September 22, 2016, I went to my first counseling session. During this session, we discussed how various illnesses develop from unresolved emotional trauma. We evaluated several of my personal relationships. This evaluation was to determine if I had any unresolved feelings and unforgiveness in my heart.

My assignments were to purchase *Healing for Damaged Emotions Workbook* by David A. Seamands and Beth Funk, to complete The 5 Love Languages Quiz by Gary Chapman, and to take a bath once a week.

As I continued to pray and attend counseling sessions, I evaluated my life. The healing (physical and emotional) process continued to manifest in my life. I continued to attend counseling as I walked through the healing process. Twice a week, I read *Scriptures for Healing* by T. L. Osborn, *A Reason for Hope Gaining* by Michael S. Barry (CTCA resource), and *Psalm 91* by Peggy Joyce Ruth. I went to sleep listening to Graham Cooke's "Healing Scriptures" on YouTube.

This routine created the opportunity for my soul and spirit to heal.

THE VICTORY & TREATMENT

Sixth Miracle Praise Report

The medical oncologist informed me that the MammaPrint test could only be completed if cancer was found. Therefore, I did not have cancer, only DCIS. DCIS develops before the first stage of cancer and is actually called stage zero.

The praise report is my body had begun to heal itself from the DCIS. The DCIS was going into remission.

The medical oncologist recommended that I receive radiation to decrease the chances of DCIS returning and/or becoming more aggressive. I was prescribed the following cream and supplement from CTCA with specific instruction: Botanicals - BCQ (CNCA), Coconut Oil, and Homeopathics - Calendula Lotion.

Family and Friend Support

My dear friend made liquefied ginger, honey, and lemon for me to drink daily. One of my spiritual mothers provided me with Alkaline water until my treatment was completed.

My work-family celebrated my life every Friday in October 2016. The first Friday in October everyone gave me either a white or pink rose and said encouraging words to me. The last Friday in October they surprised me again and provided a lunch celebration. They decorated the classroom, and the whole team wore cancer survivor bracelets.

I was truly supported and loved by many. My CSM family called and prayed with me many times and was truly a blessing.

My treatment lasted a month from Monday, November 7, 2016, to Wednesday, December 7, 2016. During this time, I was blessed to have family and friends' support.

October 29, 2016: Spiritual Reflection

During this time, I was reflecting on previous surgery recovery and my upcoming radiation treatment mentality during this season of life.

I did not want to overlook spending hours in prayer and reading my Bible daily. In 2014, I broke my right leg and did not commit to specific time in daily devotion. I wanted to spend more time in prayer this season.

Therefore, I dedicated Saturdays to prayer starting on October 29, 2016, ending on December 3, 2016. I prayed at 9 a.m., 12 p.m., and 3 p.m.

The first Saturday was awesome. God met me each time I entered into prayer. As I prayed, I realized that I was disappointed about decision I had made.

November 7, 2016 – November 11, 2016: Weekly Process and Reflection

Process
I thanked God for bringing me through the first week of radiation. Monday was a great day. Monday was my simulation. The purpose of the stimulation was to determine how to position my body for the radiation treatment. During the stimulation process, I began singing a praise and worship song. The first couple of days of treatment I felt a warm sensation on my forehead.

I discussed this feeling with the radiation oncologist. He assured me that only my right breast was receiving radiation. They had no explanation for the warm sensation on my forehead. I believed this warmness on my forehead was God giving me a sign that He was with me.

Tuesday after treatment, I felt nauseated. I ate crackers then I felt better.

Wednesday, I felt nauseated for the remainder of the day.

Thursday, I had no complications.

Friday, I felt a little nauseated. Nausea is not an uncommon side effect for a cancer patient, according to the radiation oncologist. In fact, the literature provided by CTCA listed nausea as one of the side effects of radiation. I encourage every woman and man to read the literature provided by their hospital and credible, online websites.

The quality of care that I received at CTCA was great. I appreciated all of the nurses, receptionists, radiation therapists and all of the CTCA staff. I met fabulous people who were winning the fight against cancer. I met brave people from different professions: farmers, postal workers, businessmen, and businesswomen. I knew I was there for a purpose. God led me to pray with other cancer patients. I appreciated the opportunity to pray, share my testimony, listen to their testimony, and provide words of encouragement.

Reflection

This week during prayer, I was healed emotionally. Spending time in prayer provided me the opportunity to be healed from the emotional trauma that only God could reveal.

When I reflected on this week, I realized that I never knew when I would feel physically exhausted. I appreciated my mother being there for me. She prepared dinner for me every evening after her workday. She watched me and knew when I was exhausted. I became exhausted all at once. During the radiation treatment, I found strength by singing praise and worship songs and meditating on healing scriptures.

I want to thank the following family members for attending my radiation treatments with me:

Monday - Tee Helen

Tuesday - My mother (Marilyn)

Wednesday - Tee Vera

Thursday - Tremayne

Friday - Mary

November 14, 2016 - November 18, 2016: Weekly Process and Reflection

Process

This week was an exhausting one. Monday after treatment, I stayed at my brother Matthias' place. Deciding not to drive home after treatment was a great decision. I was exhausted thirty minutes after we arrived to his place. His family showed me great hospitality. Matthias cooked delicious Chicken Tacos for dinner. The next day, I ran many personal errands.

On Tuesday morning, I drove home from Mathias's place. Then I went to work to pick up my paycheck. It was not there. Then I left to go to pick up my cousin Dwight to accompany me to my radiation appointment. My family took turns going to my appointment for moral support and transportation. This prevented me from driving after radiation therapy.

Wednesday was a hectic day. This day started with me driving to pick up my daughter-in-law. Before attending my appointment, we had to pick up my grandson's car seat and my check.

Finally, my daughter-in-law drove to CTCA. I am grateful I did not need to take her home.

Thursday, my cousin Jessica took me to my appointment. I realized I was physically exhausted from running errands from Monday to Wednesday. By the time I made it home, my energy was depleted. I slept the rest of the evening.

Friday, Matthias took me to my appointment. I enjoyed spending time with him. Matthias and my son Jonathan had an opportunity to bond. It did my heart good to hear them talk about praise and worship music over the phone. I rested for the remainder of the evening.

One day while receiving radiation, I began to sing "…miracles all around me, Holy Spirit defend me." I began to cry. The tears were rolling down my face.

Then fear grabbed my heart because I did not know if the tears would reach my treated breast area. Then I remembered that God did not give me the spirit of fear (2 Tim. 1:7). I was in the presence of the Lord and I knew He would protect me. Therefore, I resumed singing and praying.

I enjoyed talking with my sister-in-law, Faith, about her family and life experiences. Dwight was awesome. He called his siblings, and I was able to talk to all of them. That made my day. We also talked about relationships, morals, and values.

Brianna and I talked about the best communities to consider for housing. Jessica and I talked about family, my dad, growing up, and life experiences. Matthias and I talked about how we were handling life situations.

I realized I was not following the doctor's instructions because I was not exercising. I decided to follow the doctor's instructions. Therefore, I started following the Aerobic CD for exercises. I realized I was not taking care of myself.

For example, I was not drinking enough water or exercising. Self-care was important to me. I began to drink water and exercise. I started journaling and book writing. I researched how to create an app. I was disappointed in myself for my lack of consistency.

<u>Reflection</u>
During my prayer time, I realized I was not a good steward. Therefore, I repented and thanked God for allowing me to make payment arrangements with my bill collectors. I asked God to allow me to be able to honor my word. I thanked the Lord for the Ambit business opportunity that allowed me to pay my bills.

I also repented for: 1) putting my trust in my job, 2) not consistently giving my tithes and offering, 3) not being able to supply my children's needs, and 4) taking out payday loans.

After that, I asked the Lord to forgive me for falling short in these areas of my life. I also asked God to increase my faith in Him. I had bounced so many checks. Lastly, I inquired of the Lord to order my steps and bless me to be a good financial steward. God wants us to be a good steward over every area of our life.

This week I spent time with the following family members who took me to my treatment:

Monday - Faith and Naomi

Tuesday - Dwight

Wednesday - Brianna and Justin Jr.

Thursday - Jessica

Friday - Matthias

November 20, 2016 - November 23, 2016: Weekly Process and Reflection

Process

I learned my lesson from the previous week. This week, I slept through radiation. After treatments, I returned home and rested for the remainder of the day. This allowed my body to recuperate. I read the literature provided in the counseling session. Nausea decreased each week.

Periodically, I felt like fluid was behind my ears. The radiologist's assistant examined my ears stating there was no fluid present.

I also noticed my armpit skin was changing. The skin was smooth, hairless with a small skin tear. I was not informed that irritation and breakdown of skin might occur. They told me to rub a medicated cream underneath my right armpit. The therapist said I was blessed. If the irritation happened earlier, treatment would have been postponed. I continued to pray and encourage other patients.

Spending time with my family during my travel to treatment was a blessing. On Sunday, it was truly a blessing being accompanied by my brother, Ronnie. We talked about how to be an intercessor. Our conversation was inspiring.

On Monday, my cousin Carmesha went with me to my treatment. I learned so much about her. Carmesha and I met a man who was there for treatment for nine months alone. I still keep in touch with him. He is a Christian, and it was an honor to meet him. He shared his salvation story.

Seventh Miracle

We also met another man who had a conversation with us. His mother informed us that he does not talk and was overjoyed to hear her son have a conversation.

The next day Brianna, my toddler grandson Justin, and I were together. Justin ran before us into the changing room. He remembered that I had to change my clothes for treatment. He closed the door and pulled the emergency assistance button. He was instructed to open the door, and he did. While we were waiting for my name to be called for treatment, the nurse entered the waiting area and asked who needed assistance. We did not realize that Justin pulled the emergency assist alert.

On Wednesday, my toddler nephew Zechariah pressed the intercom button. The entire building heard him on the intercom. The nursing staff was looking for the baby on the intercom system. They all laughed once they found us in the waiting area. Spending time with Zechariah and his parents was a blessing. We discussed family and the Word of God.

<u>No Weekly Reflection</u>
I am grateful that the following attended my treatment appointments with me:

Sunday - Ronnie
Monday - Carmesha
Tuesday – Brianna and Justin Jr.
Wednesday - Dalonte, Lakedia, and Zecharia

November 28, 2016 - December 1, 2016, December 5, 2016:
Weekly Process and Reflection

Process

I appreciated everyone who attended this week with me. They all attended at least two or three radiation appointments with me with the exception of Mrs. Mosley. Words cannot express my gratitude. Mrs. Mosley was the only person who attended my appointment that was not a family member. I appreciated her willingness to support me during this season of my life.

The hospital staff was amazed that I had a large support team. Several of the staff informed me that I was blessed because so many patients attend their treatments alone or have only one support person. The staff began to ask, "Who is with you today?" They remembered the toddlers' names, Justin, Zechariah, and Naomi. I appreciated the hospital staff and my support team.

Reflection

During my prayer time this week, I prayed for my daughter Deja. I praised God for blessing her with a job. I asked God to guide her as she made a decision about her responsibilities.

During this week, I also forgave family members. I asked the Lord to have His way in my life and deliver me from thoughts and behaviors that are not pleasing to Him. I requested His protection. I asked Him to deliver my family from the cycle of abuse. This cycle has to be destroyed, in Jesus's Name.

I prayed, "Lord deliver me from the emotional pain of unhealthy relationships. I do not want to live my life as an angry black woman."

I had to be transparent and face my feelings. I had to move past all of the hurt, in the Name of Jesus. I prayed that the Lord would allow me to walk in victory in His precious Jesus.

I truly wanted to know where I go from here. My physical appearance was the same, but I will not be the same woman on the inside. I asked the Lord to keep me in His arms where I belong.

This week the following family members attended my appointment with me:

Monday - Mom Marilyn Burns
Tuesday - Brianna and Justin Jr.
Wednesday - Jessica
Thursday - Mom Marilyn Burns
Monday - Tommie Mosely

December 6, 2016 - December 10, 2016: Last Days of Treatment and Recovery

I do not remember the doctors, family, or friends telling me about the after effects of radiation. Praise God I have completed my radiation treatment. This week was the worst. My right breast and armpit was raw, black, and peeling. This area was a raw and open sore. I continued to apply the medicated cream and medihoney on my right breast area. These four days, I was in pain. I would not allow anything to touch my breast or armpit. I did not wear any top for these four days. I applied the cream and medihoney two to three times a day until this area began to heal. I was not expecting this to happen after radiation. I thank God for healing me from cancer.

This journey truly was a self-reflection process. I reflected on my relationships, spiritual well-being, emotions, and health.

Remember, it is important to pause and take care of yourselves. Thank you to everyone who reads my book. I pray that I have inspired, encouraged, and caused men and women to be transformed through their process.

Please listen to Graham Cooke's "Soaking Healing Scripture." This recording was very instrumental in my healing process. I also read healing scripture from the Bible.

I encourage you to accept the Lord as your personal Savior. I admitted that I was a sinner. I realized that my sin had separated me from God. I willingly turned from my sins. I believed in the death, burial, and resurrection of Jesus Christ. I accepted Jesus Christ as my personal Lord and Savior.

I encourage you to accept Him as yours. According to Romans 10:9-10, "That if thou shalt confess with thy mouth the Lord Jesus, and shalt believe in thine heart that God hath raised him from the dead, thou shalt be saved. 10 For with the heart man believeth unto righteousness; and with the mouth confession is made unto salvation," (KJV).

Prayer:

Lord, I confess my sin and ask You to forgive me of my sin. I believe in the death, burial, and resurrection of Jesus Christ. Please come into my heart, and I shall be saved.

THE WORD

Healing Scriptures:

Exodus 15:26, "And said, If thou wilt diligently hearken to the voice of the Lord thy God, and wilt do that which is right in his sight, and wilt give ear to his commandments, and keep all his statutes, I will put none of these diseases upon thee, which I have brought upon the Egyptians: for I am the Lord that healeth thee."

Exodus 23:25, "And ye shall serve the Lord your God, and he shall bless thy bread, and thy water; and I will take sickness away from the midst of thee."

Job 5:26, "Thou shalt come to thy grave in a full age, like as a shock of corn cometh in his season."

Joel 2:28, "And it shall come to pass afterward, that I will pour out my spirit upon all flesh; and your sons and your daughters shall prophesy, your old men shall dream dreams, your young men shall see visions:"

Psalms 30:2, "O Lord my God, I cried unto thee, and thou hast healed me."

Psalms 34: 7-10, "The angel of the Lord encampeth round about them that fear him, and delivereth them. O taste and see that the Lord is good: blessed is the man that trusteth in him.

O fear the Lord, ye his saints: for there is no want to them that fear him. The young lions do lack, and suffer hunger: but they that seek the Lord shall not want any good thing."

Psalm 34:19-20, "Many are the afflictions of the righteous: but the Lord delivereth him out of them all. He keepeth all his bones: not one of them is broken."

Psalm 42:11, "Why art thou cast down, O my soul? and why art thou disquieted within me? hope thou in God: for I shall yet praise him, who is the health of my countenance, and my God."

Psalms 91:14-16, "Because he hath set his love upon me, therefore will I deliver him: I will set him on high, because he hath known my name.

15 He shall call upon me, and I will answer him: I will be with him in trouble; I will deliver him, and honor him. 16 With long life will I satisfy him, and shew him my salvation."

Psalms 103: 1-6, "Bless the Lord, O my soul: and all that is within me, bless his holy name. 2 Bless the Lord, O my soul, and forget not all his benefits:

3 Who forgiveth all thine iniquities; who health all thy diseases; Who redeemeth thy life from destruction; who crowneth thee with lovingkindness and tender mercies; 5 Who satisfieth thy mouth with good things; so that thy youth is renewed like the

eagle's. 6 The Lord executeth righteousness and judgment for all that are oppressed."

Psalm 107:20, "He sent his word, and healed them, and delivered them from their destructions."

Isaiah 53:4-5, "Surely he hath borne our griefs, and carried our sorrows: yet we did esteem him stricken, smitten of God, and afflicted. 5 But he was wounded for our transgressions, he was bruised for our iniquities: the chastisement of our peace was upon him; and with his stripes we are healed."

Jeremiah 30:17, "For I will restore health unto thee, and I will heal thee of thy wounds, saith the Lord; because they called thee an Outcast, saying, This is Zion, whom no man seeketh after."

Jeremiah 33:6, "Behold, I will bring it health and cure, and I will cure them, and will reveal unto them the abundance of peace and truth."

John 6:63, "It is the spirit that quickeneth; the flesh profiteth nothing: the words that I speak unto you, they are spirit, and they are life."

I Cor. 3:16, "Know ye not that ye are the temple of God, and that the Spirit of God dwelleth in you?"

James 5:14, "And the prayer of faith shall save the sick, and the Lord shall raise him up; and if he have committed sins, they shall be forgiven him."

I Peter 2:24, "Who his own self bare our sins in his own body on the tree, that we, being dead to sins, should live unto righteousness: by whose stripes ye were healed."

I John 3:8-9, "He that committeth sin is of the devil; for the devil sinneth from the beginning. For this purpose the Son of God was manifested, that he might destroy the works of the devil. 9 Whosoever is born of God doth not commit sin; for his seed remaineth in him: and he cannot sin, because he is born of God."

FOUR GENERATION OF THE PATTERSON FAMILY

BREAST CANCER VIDEOS

To review the video on your phone, turn on your Scan QR codes feature:

Steps to set your iPhone Scan QR code:

Select the following feature:

1) Settings
2) Camera
3) Turn on the Scan QR Codes
4) Select your camera
5) Scan QR codes
6) Enjoy each video

Or view on YouTube search: The Four Generations of the Patterson Family

Patterson Family Four Generation Breast Exam Challenge

Patterson Family Four Generation Breast Cancer Awareness

Save the Girls 2018

CPSIA information can be obtained
at www.ICGtesting.com
Printed in the USA
LVHW050730140523
746938LV00010B/745